DR. BARBARA'S 7 DAYS JUICING FOR MUCUS CLEANSE

Discover natural and proven strategies for effective mucus cleanse. Full-body cleanse and detox for vitality and optimal health

Ben Hans

Table of Contents

COPYRIGHT © 2023

CHAPTER ONE

Introduction to Mucus Cleanse

Mucus cleanse, also known as mucusless diet or mucusless healing system, is a dietary approach aimed at eliminating excess mucus from the body to promote health and vitality. The concept of mucus cleanse originates from the teachings of Arnold Ehret, a German health educator, who believed that the accumulation of mucus in the body was the root cause of various ailments and diseases. The mucusless diet emphasizes the consumption of foods that are believed to leave little or no residue in the body, thus reducing mucus formation and promoting detoxification.

Historical Context and Origins

To understand the principles behind mucus cleanse, it's important to delve into its historical context and origins. Arnold Ehret, born in 1866, was a pioneering figure in the natural health movement of the early 20th century. He developed his ideas on mucusless diet after experiencing his own health struggles, which he attributed to the accumulation of mucus in his body. Ehret's teachings were influenced by various philosophical and health traditions, including naturopathy, vegetarianism, and fasting practices.

Ehret's seminal work, "The Mucusless Diet Healing System," published in 1922, outlined his dietary principles and became the cornerstone of the mucusless healing movement. In his book,

Ehret argued that the consumption of mucus-forming foods, such as meat, dairy, refined grains, and processed foods, led to the accumulation of toxic mucus in the body, which he believed was the primary cause of disease. He advocated for a diet composed mainly of fruits, leafy greens, and other non-mucus-forming foods to cleanse the body and restore health.

Principles of Mucus Cleanse

The principles of mucus cleanse are based on the idea that certain foods leave behind a mucus-like residue in the body, which can impede the body's natural detoxification processes and contribute to various health problems. According to proponents of mucus cleanse, these mucus-forming foods include animal products, dairy, refined grains, processed foods, and foods high in fat and sugar. By eliminating or reducing the consumption of these foods and focusing on whole, plant-based foods, individuals can supposedly reduce mucus production and promote detoxification.

Central to the mucus cleanse philosophy is the belief that the body has a natural ability to heal itself when provided with the right conditions. By following a mucusless diet, individuals aim to create an alkaline environment in the body, which is believed to support cellular health and vitality. Proponents of mucus cleanse also emphasize the importance of proper food combining and meal timing to optimize digestion and minimize mucus formation.

Foods to Include and Avoid

In mucus cleanse, there is a clear distinction between foods to include and foods to avoid. Proponents of the mucusless diet advocate for a predominantly plant-based diet, with an emphasis on fresh fruits, leafy greens, vegetables, nuts, seeds, and whole grains. These foods are believed to be alkaline-forming and leave minimal residues in the body, making them conducive to detoxification and health.

On the other hand, mucus-forming foods are to be avoided or minimized in mucus cleanse. These include animal products such as meat, poultry, fish, eggs, and dairy, as well as refined grains, processed foods, fried foods, and foods high in fat and sugar. Beverages such as alcohol, coffee, and sugary drinks are also discouraged, as they are believed to contribute to mucus formation and acidity in the body.

Benefits of Mucus Cleanse

Proponents of mucus cleanse claim a wide range of benefits associated with adopting a mucusless diet. These purported benefits include improved digestion, increased energy levels, clearer skin, weight loss, reduced inflammation, and enhanced overall vitality. By eliminating mucus-forming foods and promoting detoxification, individuals may experience relief from various health issues, including allergies, asthma, sinus problems, and digestive disorders.

Moreover, proponents argue that mucus cleanse can support long-term health and disease prevention by alkalizing the body and reducing the burden of toxins and metabolic waste. By nourishing the body with nutrient-dense, whole foods, individuals can support optimal cellular function and immune health, thereby reducing the risk of chronic diseases such as heart disease, diabetes, and cancer.

Criticism and Controversies

Despite its popularity in certain alternative health circles, mucus cleanse has drawn criticism and skepticism from mainstream medical professionals and nutrition experts. Critics argue that the concept of mucus cleanse lacks scientific evidence and is based on outdated theories of health and disease. While it is true that excessive mucus production can be a symptom of certain health conditions, such as respiratory infections or allergies, there is little scientific support for the idea that mucus accumulation is the root cause of disease or that specific dietary practices can eliminate mucus from the body.

Moreover, some health professionals caution against extreme dietary restrictions, such as those advocated in mucus cleanse, which may lead to nutrient deficiencies, especially in essential nutrients such as protein, calcium, vitamin B12, and omega-3 fatty acids. Restricting or eliminating entire food groups, such as animal products, can also pose challenges for certain populations, such as pregnant women, children, athletes, and individuals with specific health conditions.

Conclusion

In conclusion, mucus cleanse is a dietary approach aimed at eliminating excess mucus from the body to promote health and vitality. Rooted in the teachings of Arnold Ehret, the mucusless diet emphasizes the consumption of whole, plant-based foods while avoiding mucus-forming foods such as animal products and processed foods. Proponents claim a wide range of benefits associated with mucus cleanse, including improved digestion, increased energy, and reduced inflammation. However, the concept of mucus cleanse has drawn criticism from mainstream medical professionals due to a lack of scientific evidence and concerns about nutritional adequacy. As with any dietary approach, individuals should consult with a healthcare professional before making significant changes to their diet to ensure it meets their nutritional needs and health goals.

CHAPTER TWO

Understanding the Role of Mucus in the Body

Mucus is often misunderstood and underestimated in its importance to human health. Far from being just the sticky substance that we associate with nasal congestion or phlegm, mucus plays a vital role in various physiological processes throughout the body. In this comprehensive exploration, we will delve into the multifaceted functions of mucus, its composition, production, and its significance in maintaining homeostasis and protecting against pathogens.

Composition of Mucus

Mucus is a complex gel-like substance composed primarily of water, glycoproteins, electrolytes, and cells known as goblet cells. These goblet cells secrete mucins, large glycoproteins that give mucus its gel-like consistency and adhesive properties. Mucins contain long carbohydrate chains known as glycans, which can vary in composition and structure, influencing the viscosity and function of mucus in different tissues and organs.

In addition to mucins, mucus contains electrolytes such as sodium, potassium, and chloride, which help maintain its osmotic balance and hydration. Mucus also contains antimicrobial peptides, immunoglobulins (antibodies), enzymes, and other proteins that contribute to its antimicrobial properties and immune function.

Functions of Mucus

Mucus serves a myriad of essential functions throughout the body, including:

1. **Protection:** One of the primary functions of mucus is to protect the mucous membranes lining various organs and cavities in the body. Mucus forms a physical barrier that traps foreign particles, pathogens, and environmental toxins, preventing them from reaching underlying tissues and causing damage or infection.

2. **Moisturization:** Mucus helps keep epithelial surfaces moist and lubricated, facilitating smooth movement and preventing friction between tissues. In the respiratory system, for example, mucus moisturizes the airways, making it easier for cilia (hair-like structures) to move and clear mucus and debris from the lungs.

3. **Immune Defense:** Mucus contains various components of the immune system, including antimicrobial peptides, immunoglobulins (such as IgA), and immune cells, which help neutralize pathogens and prevent infection. Mucus also acts as a site for immune surveillance, detecting and responding to foreign invaders that breach the epithelial barrier.

4. **Respiratory Function:** In the respiratory system, mucus plays a crucial role in humidifying and filtering inhaled air, trapping

particulate matter, allergens, and pathogens. Mucus clearance mechanisms, including mucociliary clearance and coughing, help remove mucus and foreign particles from the airways, maintaining respiratory health and function.

5. **Digestive Function:** In the gastrointestinal tract, mucus lubricates and protects the lining of the stomach and intestines, facilitating the passage of food and protecting against digestive enzymes and stomach acid. Mucus also contains enzymes and bicarbonate ions that help neutralize acid and maintain an optimal pH for digestion.

6. **Reproductive Function:** In the female reproductive system, mucus produced by the cervix plays a crucial role in fertility and conception. Changes in cervical mucus consistency and composition throughout the menstrual cycle influence sperm transport and viability, facilitating fertilization and implantation.

Role of Mucus in Disease

While mucus plays a protective role in the body, dysregulation of mucus production or composition can contribute to various diseases and disorders. Excessive mucus production, as seen in conditions such as chronic bronchitis, cystic fibrosis, or asthma, can impair airflow and mucus clearance in the respiratory tract, leading to congestion, inflammation, and recurrent infections.

Conversely, insufficient mucus production or altered mucus composition can disrupt mucosal barrier function and increase susceptibility to infection and inflammation. Inflammatory bowel diseases (IBD), such as Crohn's disease and ulcerative colitis, are characterized by defects in the intestinal mucosal barrier and abnormal mucus production, contributing to chronic inflammation and tissue damage.

Conclusion

In conclusion, mucus is a versatile and indispensable substance that plays a crucial role in maintaining health and homeostasis throughout the body. From protecting mucous membranes to facilitating immune defense and maintaining respiratory and digestive function, mucus performs a myriad of essential functions essential for our well-being. Understanding the complexities of mucus composition, production, and function can provide insights into the pathophysiology of various diseases and inform the development of novel therapeutic strategies targeting mucosal health and immunity.

CHAPTER THREE

Benefits of Herbal Juicing for Mucus Cleanse

Herbal juicing has gained popularity as a natural approach to promote detoxification and support overall health and well-being. When it comes to mucus cleanse, incorporating herbal juices into your diet can offer numerous benefits, from promoting hydration and alkalization to providing essential nutrients and supporting detoxification processes. In this comprehensive exploration, we will delve into the specific benefits of herbal juicing for mucus cleanse and how different herbs can contribute to your health and vitality.

Hydration and Nutrient Absorption

One of the primary benefits of herbal juicing for mucus cleanse is hydration. Hydration is essential for maintaining the integrity and function of mucous membranes throughout the body, including the respiratory and digestive tracts. Herbal juices, made from fresh herbs and vegetables, are rich in water content, helping to keep the body hydrated and support optimal mucous membrane function.

Moreover, herbal juices are packed with essential vitamins, minerals, and phytonutrients that can be readily absorbed by the body in liquid form. This facilitates nutrient uptake and utilization, ensuring that your body receives the vital nutrients it needs to support detoxification and overall health.

Alkalization and pH Balance

Many herbs used in herbal juicing are alkaline-forming, meaning they have an alkalizing effect on the body when metabolized. Alkaline-forming foods and beverages can help counteract the acidic byproducts of metabolism and promote a more alkaline pH balance in the body. Maintaining an alkaline environment is believed to support cellular health and vitality, as well as promote detoxification and reduce inflammation.

Herbs such as kale, spinach, cucumber, parsley, and wheatgrass are commonly used in herbal juices for their alkalizing properties. These alkaline-rich herbs can help neutralize excess acidity in the body and support the body's natural detoxification processes.

Anti-inflammatory and Antioxidant Benefits

Many herbs used in herbal juicing possess potent anti-inflammatory and antioxidant properties, which can help reduce inflammation, oxidative stress, and cellular damage throughout the body. Chronic inflammation is associated with mucus production and congestion in conditions such as asthma, allergies, and sinusitis. By incorporating anti-inflammatory herbs into your herbal juices, you can help alleviate inflammation and support respiratory health.

Herbs such as ginger, turmeric, garlic, and cilantro are renowned for their anti-inflammatory and antioxidant properties. These herbs can help reduce mucus production, improve respiratory function, and support immune health, making them valuable additions to your mucus cleanse regimen.

Detoxification Support

Herbal juices can also support the body's natural detoxification processes by providing a rich source of nutrients and bioactive compounds that support liver function, digestion, and elimination. The liver plays a central role in detoxification, metabolizing toxins and waste products and facilitating their excretion from the body. Certain herbs contain compounds that can enhance liver detoxification pathways and support overall liver health.

Herbs such as dandelion, milk thistle, burdock root, and cilantro are traditionally used to support liver function and promote detoxification. These herbs can be incorporated into herbal juices to enhance their detoxifying properties and support the body's natural cleansing processes.

Immune Support

Lastly, herbal juices can provide valuable immune support, helping to strengthen the body's natural defenses against infections and pathogens. Many herbs used in herbal juicing possess immune-boosting properties, stimulating immune cell activity and enhancing immune function.

Herbs such as echinacea, elderberry, astragalus, and garlic are well-known for their immune-boosting properties. By incorporating these immune-supportive herbs into your herbal juices, you can help bolster your immune system and reduce the risk of infections, particularly during cold and flu season.

Conclusion

In conclusion, herbal juicing offers numerous benefits for mucus cleanse, from promoting hydration and alkalization to providing essential nutrients and supporting detoxification processes. By incorporating a variety of herbs into your herbal juices, you can enhance their anti-inflammatory, antioxidant, detoxifying, and immune-boosting properties, helping to promote respiratory health, reduce mucus production, and support overall well-being. Experiment with different herbal combinations to create delicious and nutritious juices that support your mucus cleanse goals and leave you feeling refreshed and revitalized.

CHAPTER FOUR

Preparing Your Body for the Cleanse

Embarking on a cleanse, such as a mucus cleanse, requires careful preparation to ensure optimal results and minimize potential discomfort. Preparing your body involves making gradual dietary and lifestyle adjustments, hydrating adequately, and setting realistic expectations for the cleanse process. In this comprehensive guide, we will explore the essential steps to prepare your body for a cleanse effectively.

Gradual Dietary Transition

Transitioning to a mucus cleanse diet abruptly can shock the body and lead to discomfort or detoxification symptoms. To minimize these effects, it's essential to make dietary changes gradually in the days leading up to the cleanse. Start by reducing or eliminating processed foods, refined sugars, caffeine, alcohol, and animal products from your diet. Instead, focus on consuming whole, plant-based foods such as fruits, vegetables, whole grains, legumes, nuts, and seeds.

Gradually increase your intake of raw fruits and vegetables, as well as herbal teas and freshly pressed juices, to prepare your body for the cleanse. This gradual transition will help acclimate your taste buds, digestive system, and metabolism to the new dietary regimen and reduce the likelihood of detoxification symptoms.

Hydration

Proper hydration is essential for supporting the body's natural detoxification processes and optimizing cleanse outcomes. Begin increasing your water intake in the days leading up to the cleanse to ensure adequate hydration. Aim to drink at least eight glasses of water per day, or more if you are physically active or live in a hot climate.

In addition to water, incorporate hydrating beverages such as herbal teas, coconut water, and freshly pressed juices into your daily routine. These beverages not only provide hydration but also deliver essential nutrients and bioactive compounds that support detoxification and overall health.

Supportive Supplements

Consider incorporating supportive supplements into your pre-cleanse regimen to prepare your body for the cleanse and enhance its detoxification capabilities. Certain supplements, such as probiotics, digestive enzymes, and herbal supplements, can help support gastrointestinal health, improve nutrient absorption, and facilitate the elimination of toxins and waste products from the body.

Probiotics, in particular, can help replenish beneficial gut bacteria and support digestive function, which is crucial for optimal nutrient absorption and elimination. Digestive enzymes can aid in the breakdown and assimilation of nutrients from food, reducing digestive discomfort and supporting overall digestive health.

Mind-Body Practices

In addition to dietary and lifestyle adjustments, incorporating mind-body practices such as meditation, yoga, deep breathing exercises, and journaling can help prepare your body and mind for the cleanse. These practices can help reduce stress, promote relaxation, and enhance mental clarity and focus, making it easier to navigate the cleanse process.

Engage in regular exercise to support lymphatic circulation, promote detoxification, and boost mood and energy levels. Choose activities that you enjoy, whether it's brisk walking, cycling, swimming, or practicing yoga. Aim for at least 30 minutes of moderate-intensity exercise most days of the week to reap the benefits for your body and mind.

Setting Realistic Expectations

Finally, it's essential to set realistic expectations for the cleanse process and understand that everyone's experience may vary. Cleansing is not a quick fix or a one-size-fits-all solution, and results may take time to manifest. Be patient and gentle with yourself throughout the cleanse journey, and listen to your body's cues and signals.

Prepare for potential detoxification symptoms such as headaches, fatigue, irritability, and digestive discomfort, especially during the initial phase of the cleanse. These symptoms are normal and may indicate that your body is releasing toxins and adjusting to the new dietary regimen. Stay hydrated, get plenty of rest, and practice self-care strategies to support your body's natural detoxification processes and minimize discomfort.

Conclusion

Preparing your body for a cleanse is a crucial step in ensuring its success and optimizing your health and well-being. By making gradual dietary transitions, prioritizing hydration, incorporating supportive supplements, engaging in mind-body practices, and setting realistic expectations, you can prepare your body and mind for the cleanse journey ahead. Listen to your body's cues, honor your unique needs and preferences, and approach the cleanse with an open mind and a spirit of self-care and self-discovery.

CHAPTER FIVE

The Seven-Day Juicing Plan: Day 1 - Detox Kickstart

Day 1 of the seven-day juicing plan marks the beginning of your journey towards cleansing and revitalizing your body. This day is designed to kickstart the detoxification process, eliminate toxins, and flood your system with essential nutrients from fresh fruits and vegetables. In this detailed guide, we will outline the juicing recipes, tips, and guidelines for Day 1 to help you embark on your cleanse journey with confidence and enthusiasm.

Morning Juice: Green Cleansing Elixir

Ingredients:

- 2 cups spinach
- 1 cucumber
- 2 stalks celery
- 1 green apple
- 1/2 lemon (peeled)
- 1-inch piece of ginger

Directions:

1. Wash all the ingredients thoroughly.

2. Cut the cucumber, celery, and apple into smaller pieces that fit your juicer chute.

3. Juice the spinach, cucumber, celery, apple, lemon, and ginger together.

4. Stir the juice well and pour it into a glass.

5. Enjoy your green cleansing elixir as soon as possible for maximum freshness and nutrient retention.

Mid-Morning Snack: Citrus Burst Juice

Ingredients:

- 2 oranges (peeled)

- 1 grapefruit (peeled)

- 1/2 lemon (peeled)

- 1 small carrot (optional)

Directions:

1. Peel the oranges, grapefruit, and lemon.

2. Cut the fruits into smaller pieces.

3. Juice the oranges, grapefruit, lemon, and carrot (if using) together.

4. Stir the juice well and pour it into a glass.

5. Savor the refreshing citrus burst juice as a mid-morning pick-me-up.

Lunch Juice: Cleansing Carrot Beet Blend

Ingredients:

- 2 large carrots

- 1 medium beet (peeled)

- 1 apple

- 1-inch piece of ginger

- 1/2 lemon (peeled)

Directions:

1. Scrub the carrots and beet thoroughly.

2. Peel the beet and cut it into smaller pieces.

3. Cut the carrots, apple, and ginger into smaller pieces.

4. Juice the carrots, beet, apple, ginger, and lemon together.

5. Mix the juice well and pour it into a glass.

6. Enjoy the vibrant and nourishing cleansing carrot beet blend as your lunch juice.

Afternoon Snack: Cooling Cucumber Mint Refresher

Ingredients:

- 1 cucumber

- 1/2 cup fresh mint leaves

- 1/2 lemon (peeled)

- 1 green apple (optional for sweetness)

Directions:

1. Wash the cucumber and mint leaves.

2. Cut the cucumber into smaller pieces.

3. Juice the cucumber, mint leaves, lemon, and apple (if using) together.

4. Stir the juice well and pour it into a glass.

5. Indulge in the cooling cucumber mint refresher as a refreshing afternoon snack.

Dinner Juice: Kale Lemon Detoxifier

Ingredients:

- 2 cups kale leaves

- 1 cucumber

- 2 stalks celery

- 1 green apple

- 1/2 lemon (peeled)

- 1-inch piece of ginger

Directions:

1. Rinse the kale leaves thoroughly.

2. Cut the cucumber, celery, and apple into smaller pieces.

3. Juice the kale, cucumber, celery, apple, lemon, and ginger together.

4. Mix the juice well and pour it into a glass.

5. Enjoy the invigorating kale lemon detoxifier as your dinner juice.

Evening Hydration: Herbal Infusion

In addition to your juices, hydrate throughout the day with plenty of water, herbal teas, and infused water. Choose herbal teas such as peppermint, chamomile, or ginger to support digestion and relaxation. Infuse water with slices of cucumber, lemon, lime, or fresh herbs for a refreshing and hydrating beverage.

Tips for Success:

1. Drink each juice slowly and mindfully, savoring the flavors and textures.

2. Stay hydrated throughout the day by drinking water and herbal teas between juices.

3. Listen to your body's cues and adjust the quantities and ingredients of the juices as needed.

4. Engage in light physical activity such as walking or yoga to support circulation and detoxification.

5. Get plenty of rest and relaxation to allow your body to rejuvenate and heal.

Conclusion: Day 1 of the seven-day juicing plan sets the stage for your cleanse journey by kickstarting the detoxification process and flooding your body with essential nutrients from fresh fruits and vegetables. By following the juicing recipes, tips, and guidelines outlined above, you can embark on your cleanse journey with enthusiasm and confidence, knowing that you are nourishing your body and supporting its natural detoxification processes. Stay committed to your goals, listen to your body's needs, and embrace the transformative power of cleansing and revitalization.

CHAPTER SIX

The Seven-Day Juicing Plan: Day 2 - Deep Cleansing

Welcome to Day 2 of your seven-day juicing plan! Today, we focus on deep cleansing to further support your body's detoxification process and promote vitality from within. With a selection of nutrient-rich juices designed to nourish your body and eliminate toxins, Day 2 will leave you feeling refreshed, revitalized, and ready to embrace the cleanse journey ahead. Let's dive into the juicing recipes, tips, and guidelines for Day 2.

Morning Juice: Detoxifying Green Goddess

Ingredients:

- 2 cups kale leaves

- 1 cucumber

- 2 stalks celery

- 1 green apple

- 1/2 lemon (peeled)

- 1-inch piece of ginger

Directions:

1. Wash the kale leaves thoroughly.

2. Cut the cucumber, celery, and apple into smaller pieces.

3. Juice the kale, cucumber, celery, apple, lemon, and ginger together.

4. Stir the juice well and pour it into a glass.

5. Start your day with the rejuvenating and detoxifying green goddess juice.

Mid-Morning Snack: Berry Blast Antioxidant Juice

Ingredients:

- 1 cup strawberries

- 1/2 cup blueberries

- 1/2 cup raspberries

- 1/2 lemon (peeled)

Directions:

1. Wash the berries thoroughly.

2. Cut the lemon into smaller pieces.

3. Juice the strawberries, blueberries, raspberries, and lemon together.

4. Mix the juice well and pour it into a glass.

5. Enjoy the antioxidant-rich berry blast juice as a mid-morning snack.

Lunch Juice: Cleansing Carrot Ginger Zinger

Ingredients:

- 3 large carrots

- 1 apple

- 1-inch piece of ginger

- 1/2 lemon (peeled)

- 1 small beet (optional)

Directions:

1. Scrub the carrots thoroughly.

2. Cut the carrots, apple, and ginger into smaller pieces.

3. Juice the carrots, apple, ginger, lemon, and beet (if using) together.

4. Stir the juice well and pour it into a glass.

5. Savor the invigorating and cleansing carrot ginger zinger as your lunch juice.

Afternoon Snack: Tropical Turmeric Delight

Ingredients:

- 1 cup pineapple chunks

- 1 small cucumber

- 1-inch piece of turmeric root (or 1/2 teaspoon ground turmeric)

- 1/2 lemon (peeled)

Directions:

1. Peel the cucumber and cut it into smaller pieces.

2. Cut the pineapple into smaller chunks.

3. Juice the pineapple, cucumber, turmeric, and lemon together.

4. Mix the juice well and pour it into a glass.

5. Indulge in the tropical turmeric delight as a refreshing afternoon snack.

Dinner Juice: Beet Greens Detoxifier

Ingredients:

- Beet greens (from 2-3 beets)

- 1 cucumber

- 2 stalks celery

- 1 green apple

- 1/2 lemon (peeled)

- Handful of parsley (optional)

Directions:

1. Wash the beet greens thoroughly.

2. Cut the cucumber, celery, and apple into smaller pieces.

3. Juice the beet greens, cucumber, celery, apple, lemon, and parsley (if using) together.

4. Stir the juice well and pour it into a glass.

5. Enjoy the vibrant and detoxifying beet greens detoxifier as your dinner juice.

Evening Hydration: Herbal Infusion

As with Day 1, hydrate throughout the day with water, herbal teas, and infused water to support hydration and detoxification. Choose herbal teas with detoxifying herbs such as dandelion, nettle, or milk thistle to further support the cleanse process.

Tips for Success:

1. Drink each juice slowly and mindfully, allowing yourself to fully experience the flavors and textures.

2. Stay hydrated throughout the day by drinking water and herbal teas between juices.

3. Incorporate light physical activity such as stretching or gentle yoga to support circulation and relaxation.

4. Listen to your body's cues and adjust the quantities and ingredients of the juices as needed to suit your preferences and needs.

5. Practice gratitude and mindfulness to cultivate a positive mindset and enhance your cleanse experience.

Conclusion: Day 2 of the seven-day juicing plan focuses on deep cleansing to support your body's detoxification process and promote vitality. By incorporating nutrient-rich juices made from fresh fruits, vegetables, and cleansing herbs, you can nourish your body from within and eliminate toxins accumulated from daily life. Embrace the transformative power of cleansing and rejuvenation as you continue your journey towards optimal health and well-being.

CHAPTER SEVEN

The Seven-Day Juicing Plan: Day 3 - Nourishment and Restoration

Day 3 of your seven-day juicing plan is all about nourishment and restoration. As you continue your cleanse journey, it's essential to replenish your body with a variety of nutrient-rich juices that support cellular renewal, enhance energy levels, and promote overall well-being. With a focus on rejuvenating ingredients and balanced flavors, Day 3 will leave you feeling refreshed, revitalized, and nourished from the inside out. Let's explore the juicing recipes, tips, and guidelines for Day 3.

Morning Juice: Sunrise Citrus Splash

Ingredients:

- 2 oranges (peeled)

- 1 grapefruit (peeled)

- 1/2 lemon (peeled)

- 1 carrot

- 1-inch piece of ginger

Directions:

1. Peel the oranges, grapefruit, and lemon.

2. Cut the carrot into smaller pieces.

3. Juice the oranges, grapefruit, lemon, carrot, and ginger together.

4. Stir the juice well and pour it into a glass.

5. Start your day with the vibrant and refreshing sunrise citrus splash juice.

Mid-Morning Snack: Green Revitalizer

Ingredients:

- 2 cups spinach

- 1 cucumber

- 1 green apple

- 1/2 lemon (peeled)

- Handful of fresh mint leaves

Directions:

1. Wash the spinach and mint leaves thoroughly.

2. Cut the cucumber and apple into smaller pieces.

3. Juice the spinach, cucumber, apple, lemon, and mint leaves together.

4. Mix the juice well and pour it into a glass.

5. Enjoy the invigorating and revitalizing green revitalizer as a mid-morning snack.

Lunch Juice: Rainbow Refresher

Ingredients:

- 1 beet (peeled)

- 1 carrot

- 1 orange (peeled)

- 1/2 lemon (peeled)

- 1-inch piece of ginger.

- Handful of kale leaves

Directions:

1. Scrub the beet and carrot thoroughly.

2. Cut the beet, carrot, and orange into smaller pieces.

3. Juice the beet, carrot, orange, lemon, ginger, and kale leaves together.

4. Stir the juice well and pour it into a glass.

5. Savor the vibrant and nutrient-packed rainbow refresher as your lunch juice.

Afternoon Snack: Berry Bliss Smoothie

Ingredients:

- 1 cup mixed berries (strawberries, blueberries, raspberries)
- 1 banana
- 1/2 cup spinach
- 1/2 cup almond milk (or any plant-based milk)
- 1 tablespoon chia seeds (optional)

Directions:

1. Wash the berries and spinach thoroughly.
2. Peel the banana and cut it into smaller pieces.
3. In a blender, combine the berries, banana, spinach, almond milk, and chia seeds (if using).
4. Blend until smooth and creamy.
5. Pour the smoothie into a glass and enjoy the delicious and nutrient-rich berry bliss smoothie as an afternoon snack.

Dinner Juice: Celery Cucumber Cooler

Ingredients:

- 3 stalks celery
- 1 cucumber
- 1 green apple

- 1/2 lemon (peeled)

- Handful of parsley

Directions:

1. Cut the celery, cucumber, and apple into smaller pieces.

2. Juice the celery, cucumber, apple, lemon, and parsley together.

3. Mix the juice well and pour it into a glass.

4. Enjoy the cooling and hydrating celery cucumber cooler as your dinner juice.

Evening Hydration: Herbal Infusion

As with previous days, hydrate throughout the day with water, herbal teas, and infused water to support hydration and promote detoxification. Choose herbal teas with calming herbs such as chamomile, lavender, or valerian root to support relaxation and restful sleep.

Tips for Success:

1. Drink each juice and smoothie slowly, allowing yourself to fully experience the flavors and textures.

2. Stay hydrated throughout the day by drinking water and herbal teas between juices and snacks.

3. Practice mindfulness and gratitude during meals to enhance your cleansing experience.

4. Incorporate light physical activity such as gentle stretching or yoga to support circulation and relaxation.

5. Listen to your body's cues and adjust the quantities and ingredients of the juices and snacks as needed to suit your preferences and needs.

Conclusion: Day 3 of the seven-day juicing plan focuses on nourishment and restoration, providing your body with a variety of nutrient-rich juices and snacks to support cellular renewal and enhance vitality. By incorporating rejuvenating ingredients and balanced flavors into your daily routine, you can replenish your body from within and continue your journey towards optimal health and well-being. Embrace the transformative power of nourishment and restoration as you continue your cleanse journey with enthusiasm and dedication.

CHAPTER EIGHT

The Seven-Day Juicing Plan: Day 4 - Rejuvenation

Day 4 of your seven-day juicing plan is dedicated to rejuvenation, focusing on refreshing your body and mind with a selection of revitalizing juices and nourishing snacks. As you progress through the cleanse journey, Day 4 provides an opportunity to replenish your energy levels, promote mental clarity, and support overall well-being. Let's explore the juicing recipes, tips, and guidelines for Day 4 to help you embrace rejuvenation and vitality.

Morning Juice: Energizing Green Detox

Ingredients:

- 2 cups spinach

- 1 cucumber

- 2 stalks celery

- 1 green apple

- 1/2 lemon (peeled)

- 1-inch piece of ginger

Directions:

1. Wash the spinach thoroughly.

2. Cut the cucumber, celery, and apple into smaller pieces.

3. Juice the spinach, cucumber, celery, apple, lemon, and ginger together.

4. Stir the juice well and pour it into a glass.

5. Start your day with the energizing green detox juice to boost your energy levels and support detoxification.

Mid-Morning Snack: Berry Banana Smoothie

Ingredients:

- 1 cup mixed berries (strawberries, blueberries, raspberries)

- 1 banana

- 1/2 cup spinach

- 1/2 cup almond milk (or any plant-based milk)

- 1 tablespoon almond butter (optional)

Directions:

1. Wash the berries and spinach thoroughly.

2. Peel the banana and cut it into smaller pieces.

3. In a blender, combine the berries, banana, spinach, almond milk, and almond butter (if using).

4. Blend until smooth and creamy.

5. Pour the smoothie into a glass and enjoy the delicious and nourishing berry banana smoothie as a mid-morning snack.

Lunch Juice: Citrus Beet Blast

Ingredients:

- 1 beet (peeled)
- 1 orange (peeled)
- 1/2 grapefruit (peeled)
- 1 carrot
- 1/2 lemon (peeled)
- 1-inch piece of ginger

Directions:

1. Scrub the beet and carrot thoroughly.

2. Cut the beet, orange, grapefruit, and carrot into smaller pieces.

3. Juice the beet, orange, grapefruit, carrot, lemon, and ginger together.

4. Stir the juice well and pour it into a glass.

5. Savor the refreshing and rejuvenating citrus beet blast as your lunch juice.

Afternoon Snack: Green Goddess Avocado Dip

Ingredients:

- 1 ripe avocado

- Handful of fresh spinach or kale

- 1/2 lemon (juiced)

- 1 clove garlic (optional)

- Pinch of sea salt

- Dash of cayenne pepper (optional)

Directions:

1. Scoop the flesh of the avocado into a blender or food processor.

2. Add the fresh spinach or kale, lemon juice, garlic (if using), sea salt, and cayenne pepper (if using).

3. Blend until smooth and creamy.

4. Transfer the dip to a bowl and serve with raw vegetable sticks or whole grain crackers.

5. Enjoy the nourishing and revitalizing green goddess avocado dip as an afternoon snack.

Dinner Juice: Tropical Turmeric Twist

Ingredients:

- 1 cup pineapple chunks

- 1 cucumber

- 1-inch piece of turmeric root (or 1/2 teaspoon ground turmeric)

- 1/2 lemon (peeled)

- Handful of cilantro

Directions:

1. Peel the cucumber.

2. Cut the pineapple into smaller chunks.

3. Juice the pineapple, cucumber, turmeric, lemon, and cilantro together.

4. Mix the juice well and pour it into a glass.

5. Indulge in the tropical turmeric twist as your dinner juice.

Evening Hydration: Herbal Infusion

As with previous days, hydrate throughout the day with water, herbal teas, and infused water to support hydration and promote detoxification. Choose herbal teas with relaxing herbs such as lavender, chamomile, or passionflower to support relaxation and restful sleep.

Tips for Success:

1. Drink each juice, smoothie, and snack slowly and mindfully, allowing yourself to fully savor the flavors and textures.

2. Stay hydrated throughout the day by drinking water and herbal teas between juices and snacks.

3. Incorporate mindfulness practices such as deep breathing or meditation to promote relaxation and reduce stress.

4. Engage in light physical activity such as gentle stretching or walking to support circulation and rejuvenation.

5. Listen to your body's cues and adjust the quantities and ingredients of the juices and snacks as needed to suit your preferences and needs.

Conclusion: Day 4 of the seven-day juicing plan focuses on rejuvenation, providing your body with a variety of revitalizing juices and nourishing snacks to replenish your energy levels and promote overall well-being. By incorporating nutrient-rich ingredients and balanced flavors into your daily routine, you can embrace rejuvenation and vitality as you continue your cleanse journey with enthusiasm and dedication. Embrace the transformative power of nourishment and restoration as you nourish your body and mind from within.

CHAPTER NINE

The Seven-Day Juicing Plan: Day 5 - Revitalization

Day 5 of your seven-day juicing plan focuses on revitalization, providing your body with a variety of rejuvenating juices and snacks to promote energy, vitality, and overall well-being. As you continue your cleanse journey, Day 5 offers an opportunity to revitalize your body and mind, supporting detoxification and renewal from within. Let's explore the juicing recipes, tips, and guidelines for Day 5 to help you embrace revitalization and feel refreshed and invigorated.

Morning Juice: Green Energy Boost

Ingredients:

- 2 cups kale leaves

- 1 cucumber

- 2 stalks celery

- 1 green apple

- 1/2 lemon (peeled)

- 1-inch piece of ginger

Directions:

1. Wash the kale leaves thoroughly.

2. Cut the cucumber, celery, and apple into smaller pieces.

3. Juice the kale, cucumber, celery, apple, lemon, and ginger together.

4. Stir the juice well and pour it into a glass.

5. Start your day with the energizing green energy boost juice to kickstart your morning with vitality.

Mid-Morning Snack: Berry Beet Blast Smoothie

Ingredients:

- 1/2 cup mixed berries (strawberries, blueberries, raspberries)

- 1/2 cup cooked beet chunks (cooled)

- 1/2 cup spinach

- 1 banana

- 1/2 cup almond milk (or any plant-based milk)

- 1 tablespoon hemp seeds (optional)

Directions:

1. Wash the berries and spinach thoroughly.

2. Cook the beet until tender, then allow it to cool.

3. Peel the banana and cut it into smaller pieces.

4. In a blender, combine the berries, cooked beet chunks, spinach, banana, almond milk, and hemp seeds (if using).

5. Blend until smooth and creamy.

6. Pour the smoothie into a glass and enjoy the delicious and nourishing berry beet blast smoothie as a mid-morning snack.

Lunch Juice: Citrus Carrot Glow

Ingredients:

- 3 large carrots

- 1 orange (peeled)

- 1/2 grapefruit (peeled)

- 1/2 lemon (peeled)

- 1-inch piece of ginger

- Handful of parsley

Directions:

1. Scrub the carrots thoroughly.

2. Cut the carrots, orange, and grapefruit into smaller pieces.

3. Juice the carrots, orange, grapefruit, lemon, ginger, and parsley together.

4. Stir the juice well and pour it into a glass.

5. Savor the refreshing and revitalizing citrus carrot glow as your lunch juice.

Afternoon Snack: Tropical Green Smoothie

Ingredients:

- 1 cup pineapple chunks

- 1/2 cup mango chunks

- 1/2 cup spinach

- 1/2 cup coconut water

- 1 tablespoon chia seeds (optional)

Directions:

1. Wash the spinach thoroughly.

2. Cut the pineapple and mango into smaller chunks.

3. In a blender, combine the pineapple, mango, spinach, coconut water, and chia seeds (if using).

4. Blend until smooth and creamy.

5. Pour the smoothie into a glass and enjoy the tropical green smoothie as an afternoon snack.

Dinner Juice: Beetroot Detoxifier

Ingredients:

- 2 medium beets (peeled)

- 1 cucumber

- 2 stalks celery

- 1 green apple

- 1/2 lemon (peeled)

- Handful of cilantro

Directions:

1. Scrub the beets thoroughly and peel them.

2. Cut the cucumber, celery, and apple into smaller pieces.

3. Juice the beets, cucumber, celery, apple, lemon, and cilantro together.

4. Mix the juice well and pour it into a glass.

5. Enjoy the vibrant and detoxifying beetroot detoxifier as your dinner juice.

Evening Hydration: Herbal Infusion

As with previous days, hydrate throughout the day with water, herbal teas, and infused water to support hydration and promote detoxification. Choose herbal teas with invigorating herbs such as peppermint, ginger, or lemon balm to refresh your body and mind.

Tips for Success:

1. Drink each juice, smoothie, and snack slowly and mindfully, allowing yourself to fully savor the flavors and textures.

2. Stay hydrated throughout the day by drinking water and herbal teas between juices and snacks.

3. Incorporate relaxation techniques such as deep breathing or gentle stretching to promote relaxation and reduce stress.

4. Listen to your body's cues and adjust the quantities and ingredients of the juices and snacks as needed to suit your preferences and needs.

5. Practice gratitude and mindfulness to cultivate a positive mindset and enhance your cleansing experience.

Conclusion: Day 5 of the seven-day juicing plan focuses on revitalization, providing your body with a variety of rejuvenating juices and snacks to promote energy, vitality, and overall well-being. By incorporating nutrient-rich ingredients and balanced flavors into your daily routine, you can embrace revitalization and feel refreshed and invigorated as you continue your cleanse journey with enthusiasm and dedication. Embrace the transformative power of nourishment and renewal as you nourish your body and mind from within.

CHAPTER TEN

The Seven-Day Juicing Plan: Day 6 - Inner Balance and Harmony

Day 6 of your seven-day juicing plan is dedicated to achieving inner balance and harmony, focusing on nurturing both your body and mind with a selection of calming and grounding juices and snacks. As you approach the end of your cleanse journey, Day 6 offers an opportunity to reconnect with yourself, promote emotional well-being, and cultivate a sense of inner peace. Let's explore the juicing recipes, tips, and guidelines for Day 6 to help you embrace inner balance and harmony.

Morning Juice: Calming Green Goddess

Ingredients:

- 2 cups spinach
- 1 cucumber
- 2 stalks celery
- 1 green apple
- 1/2 lemon (peeled)
- 1-inch piece of ginger
- Handful of fresh mint leaves

Directions:

1. Wash the spinach and mint leaves thoroughly.

2. Cut the cucumber, celery, and apple into smaller pieces.

3. Juice the spinach, cucumber, celery, apple, lemon, ginger, and mint leaves together.

4. Stir the juice well and pour it into a glass.

5. Start your day with the calming green goddess juice to promote inner balance and harmony.

Mid-Morning Snack: Creamy Avocado Dip with Vegetable Crudites

Ingredients for Avocado Dip:

- 1 ripe avocado

- 1/2 lemon (juiced)

- 1 clove garlic (optional)

- Pinch of sea salt

Ingredients for Vegetable Crudites:

- Assorted raw vegetables (carrots, cucumber, bell peppers, celery, etc.)

Directions:

1. Scoop the flesh of the avocado into a bowl.

2. Mash the avocado with a fork until creamy.

3. Add the lemon juice, garlic (if using), and sea salt to the mashed avocado and mix well.

4. Prepare the raw vegetables by washing and cutting them into sticks or bite-sized pieces.

5. Serve the avocado dip alongside the vegetable crudites for a nourishing and balanced mid-morning snack.

Lunch Juice: Harmony Beet Blend

Ingredients:

- 2 medium beets (peeled)

- 1 carrot

- 1 orange (peeled)

- 1/2 lemon (peeled)

- 1-inch piece of ginger

- Handful of parsley

Directions:

1. Scrub the beets thoroughly and peel them.

2. Cut the carrot and orange into smaller pieces.

3. Juice the beets, carrot, orange, lemon, ginger, and parsley together.

4. Stir the juice well and pour it into a glass.

5. Savor the harmonizing and grounding beet blend as your lunch juice.

Afternoon Snack: Serenity Berry Smoothie Bowl

Ingredients:

- 1 frozen banana

- 1/2 cup mixed berries (strawberries, blueberries, raspberries)

- 1/2 cup almond milk (or any plant-based milk)

- 1 tablespoon chia seeds

- Toppings: sliced banana, berries, shredded coconut, granola, etc.

Directions:

1. In a blender, combine the frozen banana, mixed berries, almond milk, and chia seeds.

2. Blend until smooth and creamy, adding more almond milk if needed to achieve desired consistency.

3. Pour the smoothie into a bowl.

4. Top with sliced banana, additional berries, shredded coconut, granola, or your favorite toppings.

5. Enjoy the serenity berry smoothie bowl as a nourishing and satisfying afternoon snack.

Dinner Juice: Zen Cucumber Cooler

Ingredients:

- 2 cucumbers

- 2 stalks celery

- 1 green apple

- 1/2 lemon (peeled)

- Handful of fresh basil leaves

Directions:

1. Wash the cucumbers and basil leaves thoroughly.

2. Cut the cucumbers, celery, and apple into smaller pieces.

3. Juice the cucumbers, celery, apple, lemon, and basil leaves together.

4. Mix the juice well and pour it into a glass.

5. Indulge in the refreshing and calming zen cucumber cooler as your dinner juice.

Evening Hydration: Herbal Infusion

As with previous days, hydrate throughout the day with water, herbal teas, and infused water to support hydration and promote relaxation. Choose herbal teas with soothing herbs such as chamomile, lavender, or lemon balm to enhance your sense of inner peace and tranquility.

Tips for Success:

1. Drink each juice, smoothie, and snack slowly and mindfully, savoring the flavors and textures.

2. Practice deep breathing or meditation to promote relaxation and reduce stress.

3. Spend time in nature or engage in activities that bring you joy and serenity.

4. Reflect on your cleanse journey and express gratitude for the opportunity to nurture your body and mind.

5. Listen to your body's cues and honor your need for rest and relaxation as you approach the end of the cleanse.

Conclusion: Day 6 of the seven-day juicing plan focuses on achieving inner balance and harmony, nurturing both your body and mind with calming and grounding juices and snacks. By incorporating nourishing ingredients and mindful practices into your daily routine, you can promote emotional well-being, cultivate a sense of inner peace, and embrace the transformative power of self-care and self-discovery. As you continue your cleanse journey, remember to prioritize self-care, listen to your body's needs, and embrace the journey with openness and gratitude.

DAY 7

Morning Juice: Soothing Green Elixir Ingredients:

- 2 cups spinach
- 1 cucumber
- 2 stalks celery
- 1 green apple
- 1/2 lemon (peeled)
- 1-inch piece of ginger
- Handful of fresh cilantro leaves

Directions:

1. Wash the spinach and cilantro leaves thoroughly.

2. Cut the cucumber, celery, and apple into smaller pieces.

3. Juice the spinach, cucumber, celery, apple, lemon, ginger, and cilantro together.

4. Stir the juice well and pour it into a glass.

5. Start your day with the soothing green elixir to promote inner balance and harmony.

Mid-Morning Snack: Creamy Coconut Yogurt with Berries
Ingredients:

- 1 cup coconut yogurt

- 1/2 cup mixed berries (blueberries, strawberries, raspberries)

- 1 tablespoon honey or maple syrup (optional)

- Sprinkle of cinnamon (optional)

Directions:

1. Spoon the coconut yogurt into a bowl.

2. Add the mixed berries on top.

3. Drizzle with honey or maple syrup and sprinkle with cinnamon if desired.

4. Enjoy the creamy coconut yogurt with berries as a refreshing mid-morning snack.

Lunch Juice: Cleansing Carrot Citrus Fusion Ingredients:

- 3 carrots

- 1 orange (peeled)

- 1/2 lemon (peeled)

- 1-inch piece of turmeric root

- Handful of fresh mint leaves

Directions:

1. Scrub the carrots and peel the lemon and orange.

2. Cut the carrots into smaller pieces.

3. Juice the carrots, orange, lemon, turmeric, and mint leaves together.

4. Stir the juice well and pour it into a glass.

5. Savor the cleansing carrot citrus fusion as your lunch juice.

Afternoon Snack: Cooling Cucumber Gazpacho Ingredients:

- 2 cucumbers

- 1 ripe avocado

- 1/2 lime (juiced)

- 1/4 cup fresh cilantro leaves

- Pinch of sea salt and black pepper

- Optional: diced tomatoes, red onion, jalapeño for garnish

Directions:

1. Peel and chop one cucumber, and reserve the other for garnish.

2. In a blender, combine the chopped cucumber, avocado, lime juice, cilantro leaves, sea salt, and black pepper.

3. Blend until smooth and creamy.

4. Chill the gazpacho in the refrigerator for at least 30 minutes.

5. Serve the gazpacho in bowls, garnished with diced cucumber, tomatoes, red onion, and jalapeño if desired.

Dinner Juice: Relaxing Lemon Ginger Zinger Ingredients:

- 2 apples
- 1 lemon (peeled)
- 1-inch piece of ginger
- 1/2 fennel bulb
- Handful of fresh basil leaves

Directions:

1. Cut the apples and lemon into smaller pieces.

2. Juice the apples, lemon, ginger, fennel, and basil leaves together.

3. Mix the juice well and pour it into a glass.

4. Indulge in the relaxing lemon ginger zinger as your dinner juice.

Evening Hydration: Herbal Infusion As with previous days, hydrate throughout the day with water, herbal teas, and infused water to support hydration and promote relaxation. Choose herbal teas with soothing herbs such as chamomile, peppermint, or ginger to enhance your sense of inner peace and tranquility.

Tips for Success:

1. Drink each juice, snack, and infusion slowly and mindfully, focusing on the sensations it brings to your body.

2. Practice deep breathing or meditation to promote relaxation and reduce stress.

3. Spend time in quiet reflection or engage in gentle movement exercises like yoga or walking.

4. Listen to your body's signals and adjust the cleanse plan as needed to suit your individual needs and preferences.

5. Express gratitude for the opportunity to nourish your body and mind with healing foods and practices.

CHAPTER 11

SOME HERBAL JUICE RECIPES FOR MUCUS CLEANSE

1. **Peppermint and Lemon Juice**

   - **Definition:** Peppermint and lemon juice is a refreshing blend known for its ability to clear congestion and soothe irritated throats.

   - **Ingredients:** Fresh peppermint leaves, lemon juice, water, honey (optional).

- **How to Prepare:** Blend fresh peppermint leaves with lemon juice and water. Strain the mixture and add honey if desired.

- **How to Use:** Consume a small glass of this juice daily on an empty stomach.

- **Dosage:** 1 glass per day.

- **Side Effects:** Peppermint may cause heartburn in some individuals.

- **Precautions:** Avoid if you have gastroesophageal reflux disease (GERD).

2. Ginger and Turmeric Juice

- **Definition:** Ginger and turmeric juice is renowned for its anti-inflammatory properties, making it effective in reducing mucus buildup.

- **Ingredients:** Fresh ginger root, fresh turmeric root, lemon juice, water, honey (optional).

- **How to Prepare:** Blend ginger and turmeric roots with lemon juice and water. Strain the mixture and sweeten with honey if desired.

- **How to Use:** Consume a small glass of this juice daily.

- **Dosage:** 1 glass per day.

- **Side Effects:** May cause stomach upset or heartburn in some individuals.

- **Precautions:** Avoid if you have gallbladder issues or are on blood-thinning medications.

3. Lemon and Honey Tea

- **Definition:** Lemon and honey tea is a classic remedy for soothing sore throats and reducing mucus production.

- **Ingredients:** Lemon juice, honey, hot water.

- **How to Prepare:** Mix lemon juice and honey in hot water until dissolved.

- **How to Use:** Drink this tea multiple times a day, especially during cold or flu.

- **Dosage:** As needed.

- **Side Effects:** None when consumed in moderation.

- **Precautions:** Avoid if allergic to citrus fruits or honey.

4. Eucalyptus and Orange Juice

- **Definition:** Eucalyptus and orange juice is a refreshing blend that can help clear nasal passages and reduce mucus.

- **Ingredients:** Fresh eucalyptus leaves, fresh orange juice.

- **How to Prepare:** Blend eucalyptus leaves with orange juice.

- **How to Use:** Consume a small glass of this juice daily.

- **Dosage:** 1 glass per day.

- **Side Effects:** Eucalyptus oil can be toxic if ingested in large quantities.

- **Precautions:** Use only small amounts of eucalyptus leaves and avoid the oil.

5. Pineapple and Celery Juice

- **Definition:** Pineapple and celery juice is rich in bromelain and antioxidants, which can help break down mucus and alleviate congestion.

- **Ingredients:** Fresh pineapple chunks, celery stalks, water.

- **How to Prepare:** Blend pineapple and celery with water until smooth.

- **How to Use:** Consume a small glass of this juice daily.

- **Dosage:** 1 glass per day.

- **Side Effects:** None when consumed in moderation.

- **Precautions:** Celery may cause allergic reactions in some individuals.

6. Garlic and Lemon Juice

- **Definition:** Garlic and lemon juice is a potent combination known for its immune-boosting and mucus-clearing properties.

- **Ingredients:** Fresh garlic cloves, lemon juice, water, honey (optional).

- **How to Prepare:** Blend garlic cloves with lemon juice and water. Strain the mixture and sweeten with honey if desired.

- **How to Use:** Consume a small glass of this juice daily.

- **Dosage:** 1 glass per day.

- **Side Effects:** Garlic may cause bad breath and digestive upset in some individuals.

- **Precautions:** Avoid if allergic to garlic or citrus fruits.

7. Nettle and Lemon Juice

- **Definition:** Nettle and lemon juice is a detoxifying blend that can help reduce inflammation and mucus production.

- **Ingredients:** Fresh nettle leaves, lemon juice, water, honey (optional).

- **How to Prepare:** Blend nettle leaves with lemon juice and water. Strain the mixture and sweeten with honey if desired.

- **How to Use:** Consume a small glass of this juice daily.

- **Dosage:** 1 glass per day.

- **Side Effects:** Nettle may cause allergic reactions in some individuals.

- **Precautions:** Handle nettle leaves with gloves to avoid skin irritation.

8. Apple Cider Vinegar and Honey Tonic

- **Definition:** Apple cider vinegar and honey tonic is a popular remedy for boosting immunity and breaking down mucus.

- **Ingredients:** Apple cider vinegar, honey, warm water.

- **How to Prepare:** Mix apple cider vinegar and honey in warm water until dissolved.

- **How to Use:** Drink this tonic once daily.

- **Dosage:** 1 serving per day.

- **Side Effects:** Apple cider vinegar may erode tooth enamel and cause throat irritation if not diluted.

- **Precautions:** Dilute vinegar properly and rinse mouth after consumption.

9. Cayenne Pepper and Lemon Juice

- **Definition:** Cayenne pepper and lemon juice is a spicy blend that can help clear sinuses and reduce mucus production.

- **Ingredients:** Cayenne pepper powder, lemon juice, warm water, honey (optional).

- **How to Prepare:** Mix cayenne pepper powder and lemon juice in warm water. Sweeten with honey if desired.

- **How to Use:** Drink this mixture once daily.

- **Dosage:** 1 serving per day.

- **Side Effects:** Cayenne pepper may cause stomach irritation in some individuals.

- **Precautions:** Use in moderation, especially if sensitive to spicy foods.

10. Fenugreek and Honey Tea

- **Definition:** Fenugreek and honey tea is a soothing blend that can help alleviate respiratory congestion and thin mucus.

- **Ingredients:** Fenugreek seeds, honey, hot water.

- **How to Prepare:** Steep fenugreek seeds in hot water for 10 minutes. Strain and add honey.

- **How to Use:** Drink this tea 2-3 times a day.

- **Dosage:** As needed.

- **Side Effects:** Fenugreek may cause digestive upset in some individuals.

- **Precautions:** Avoid if pregnant or allergic to fenugreek.

11. **Lemon Balm and Chamomile Tea**

- **Definition:** Lemon balm and chamomile tea is a calming blend that can help reduce inflammation and mucus production.

- **Ingredients:** Lemon balm leaves, chamomile flowers, hot water, honey (optional).

- **How to Prepare:** Steep lemon balm leaves and chamomile flowers in hot water for 5-10 minutes. Sweeten with honey if desired.

- **How to Use:** Drink this tea 2-3 times a day.

- **Dosage:** As needed.

- **Side Effects:** None when consumed in moderation.

- **Precautions:** Avoid if allergic to plants in the Asteraceae family.

12.   **Horseradish and Lemon Juice**

- **Definition:** Horseradish and lemon juice is a potent blend that can help clear congested sinuses and loosen mucus.

- **Ingredients:** Fresh horseradish root, lemon juice, water, honey (optional).

- **How to Prepare:** Blend horseradish root with lemon juice and water. Strain and sweeten with honey if desired.

- **How to Use:** Consume a small glass of this juice daily.

- **Dosage:** 1 glass per day.

- **Side Effects:** Horseradish may cause stomach upset or irritation in some individuals.

- **Precautions:** Use in small amounts and avoid if sensitive to spicy foods.

13.   **Dandelion and Ginger Tea**

- **Definition:** Dandelion and ginger tea is a detoxifying blend that can help reduce mucus production and support liver function.

- **Ingredients:** Dandelion root, fresh ginger root, hot water, honey (optional).

- **How to Prepare:** Steep dandelion root and ginger in hot water for 10-15 minutes. Sweeten with honey if desired.

- **How to Use:** Drink this tea 2-3 times a day.

- **Dosage:** As needed.

- **Side Effects:** Dandelion may cause allergic reactions in some individuals.

- **Precautions:** Avoid if allergic to plants in the Asteraceae family.

14. **Rosemary and Thyme Infusion**

- **Definition:** Rosemary and thyme infusion is a fragrant blend that can help clear congestion and soothe respiratory discomfort.

- **Ingredients:** Fresh rosemary sprigs, fresh thyme sprigs, hot water, honey (optional).

- **How to Prepare:** Steep rosemary and thyme in hot water for 10-15 minutes. Sweeten with honey if desired.

- **How to Use:** Drink this infusion 2-3 times a day.

- **Dosage:** As needed.

- **Side Effects:** None when consumed in moderation.

- **Precautions:** Avoid if pregnant or allergic to rosemary or thyme.

15.   **Sage and Lemon Juice**

- **Definition:** Sage and lemon juice is a soothing blend that can help reduce mucus production and calm respiratory inflammation.

- **Ingredients:** Fresh sage leaves, lemon juice, water, honey (optional).

- **How to Prepare:** Blend sage leaves with lemon juice and water. Strain and sweeten with honey if desired.

- **How to Use:** Consume a small glass of this juice daily.

- **Dosage:** 1 glass per day.

- **Side Effects:** Sage may cause digestive upset in some individuals.

- **Precautions:** Avoid if pregnant or breastfeeding.

SOME HERBAL REMEDIES YOU SHOULD KNOW

Eucalyptus:

Definition: Eucalyptus refers to a genus of flowering trees and shrubs, primarily native to Australia but also found in other parts of the world. Eucalyptus essential oil, extracted from the leaves of certain species, has a long history of use in traditional medicine for its potential health benefits.

Ingredients: Eucalyptus essential oil contains various bioactive compounds, including eucalyptol (cineole), terpenes, and flavonoids. These compounds are believed to contribute to the oil's medicinal properties, including its potential as an expectorant, decongestant, antiseptic, and anti-inflammatory.

How to Prepare: Eucalyptus essential oil can be used in aromatherapy, diffused in the air, or diluted and applied topically to the skin. It can also be added to steam inhalations or chest rubs to help relieve respiratory symptoms.

Dosage: The appropriate dosage of eucalyptus essential oil can vary depending on factors such as age, health status, and the specific application being used. It's important to follow the recommended dosage on the product label or consult with a qualified aromatherapist or healthcare professional for personalized guidance.

How to Use: Eucalyptus essential oil can be used aromatically, topically, or internally, depending on the intended application. It's often used to alleviate respiratory congestion, soothe sore muscles, promote relaxation, and support overall well-being.

Side Effects: Eucalyptus essential oil is generally considered safe for most people when used appropriately. However, it can be toxic if ingested in large amounts and should not be applied directly to the skin without proper dilution. Some individuals may experience allergic reactions or respiratory irritation when exposed to eucalyptus oil. It's important to use eucalyptus oil with caution, especially around children and pets. Pregnant or breastfeeding individuals should consult with a healthcare professional before using eucalyptus oil. If any adverse effects occur, discontinue use and seek medical attention.

Feverfew:

Definition: Feverfew, scientifically known as Tanacetum parthenium, is a perennial herb native to Europe but also found in other parts of the world. It has a long history of use in traditional medicine, particularly in European folk medicine, for its potential health benefits.

Ingredients: Feverfew contains various bioactive compounds, including sesquiterpene lactones (such as parthenolide), flavonoids, and volatile oils. These compounds are believed to contribute to the herb's medicinal properties, including its potential as an anti-inflammatory, analgesic, and migraine prophylactic.

How to Prepare: Feverfew is typically consumed as an herbal tea, tincture, or in supplement form (such as capsules or tablets). To make tea, dried feverfew leaves and flowers are steeped in hot water for several minutes before being strained and consumed.

Dosage: The appropriate dosage of feverfew can vary depending on factors such as age, health status, and the specific preparation being used. It's important to follow the recommended dosage on the product label or consult with a qualified herbalist or healthcare professional for personalized guidance.

How to Use: Feverfew tea, tincture, or supplements are typically taken orally. It's often used to alleviate headaches, including migraines, and to support overall well-being.

Side Effects: Feverfew is generally considered safe for most people when used in moderate amounts. However, some individuals may experience mild side effects such as gastrointestinal upset or allergic reactions. It may also interact with certain medications or have adverse effects in individuals with certain health conditions, such as bleeding disorders or pregnancy. It's important to use feverfew under the guidance of a healthcare professional and to discontinue use if any adverse effects occur.

Bio Ferro Tonic:

Definition: Bio Ferro Tonic is a dietary supplement primarily composed of herbs and minerals. It's often marketed as a natural way to support overall health, particularly by promoting blood health and circulation.

Ingredients: Typical ingredients in Bio Ferro Tonic may include a blend of herbs such as burdock root, yellow dock root, sarsaparilla root, and cascara sagrada bark, along with minerals like iron and potassium phosphate.

How to Prepare: Bio Ferro Tonic usually comes in liquid form and is typically taken orally. It's important to follow the instructions on the product label for dosage and administration.

Dosage: The dosage can vary depending on the specific product and individual needs. It's crucial to consult with a healthcare professional or follow the recommended dosage on the product label to avoid potential side effects.

How to Use: Bio Ferro Tonic is often taken by adding the recommended dosage to water or juice and consuming it orally. It's important to shake the bottle well before use and store it according to the manufacturer's instructions.

Side Effects: While Bio Ferro Tonic is generally considered safe when used as directed, some individuals may experience side effects such as digestive discomfort, allergic reactions, or interactions with medications. It's essential to consult with a healthcare provider before starting any new supplement regimen, especially if you have underlying health conditions or are taking medications.

Bladderwrack:

Definition: Bladderwrack is a type of seaweed or marine algae commonly used in traditional medicine and as a dietary supplement. It's known for its potential health benefits, particularly related to thyroid health and weight management.

Ingredients: Bladderwrack contains various nutrients, including iodine, vitamins, minerals, and antioxidants. The primary active components are iodine and fucoidan, a type of carbohydrate found in brown seaweeds.

How to Prepare: Bladderwrack supplements are available in various forms, including capsules, powders, and liquid extracts. They can be taken orally with water or added to smoothies and other beverages.

Dosage: The appropriate dosage of bladderwrack can vary based on factors such as age, health status, and the specific product being used. It's essential to follow the recommended dosage on the product label or consult with a healthcare professional for personalized guidance.

How to Use: Bladderwrack supplements are typically taken orally, either with water or mixed into food or beverages. It's important to follow the instructions on the product label and avoid exceeding the recommended dosage.

Side Effects: While bladderwrack is generally considered safe for most people when used in moderation, excessive intake of iodine from bladderwrack supplements can cause thyroid dysfunction and other adverse effects. Individuals with thyroid disorders, iodine sensitivity, or certain medical conditions should exercise caution and consult with a healthcare provider before using bladderwrack supplements. Common side effects may include digestive upset, allergic reactions, or interactions with medications.

Burdock:

Definition: Burdock, scientifically known as Arctium lappa, is a biennial plant native to Europe and Asia but now found worldwide. It's part of the Asteraceae family and has been used for centuries in traditional medicine and culinary practices.

Ingredients: Burdock contains various nutrients, including carbohydrates, fiber, vitamins (such as vitamin B6, folate, and vitamin C), and minerals (including potassium, magnesium, and manganese). It also contains active compounds such as polyphenols and volatile oils.

How to Prepare: Burdock can be prepared and consumed in various ways. The roots, leaves, and seeds are all utilized for different purposes. The root is commonly used in cooking, herbal teas, tinctures, and supplements, while the leaves and seeds are sometimes used in herbal preparations.

Dosage: The appropriate dosage of burdock root can vary depending on the specific form and intended use. For culinary purposes, there are no strict dosage guidelines, but for supplements or herbal remedies, it's essential to follow the recommended dosage on the product label or consult with a healthcare professional.

How to Use: Burdock root can be used in cooking by peeling, slicing, and adding it to soups, stews, stir-fries, or salads. It can also be brewed into a tea or used to make tinctures or extracts for medicinal purposes. Some people may also take burdock root supplements in capsule or powder form.

Side Effects: While burdock is generally considered safe for most people when consumed in moderate amounts, some individuals may experience allergic reactions or digestive upset. Additionally, burdock may interact with certain medications or have adverse effects in individuals with certain health conditions, such as diabetes or allergies to plants in the Asteraceae family. It's important to consult with a healthcare provider before using burdock, especially if you have underlying health conditions or are taking medications.

Cascara Sagrada:

Definition: Cascara Sagrada, scientifically known as Rhamnus purshiana, is a species of buckthorn native to western North America. It has been used traditionally as a laxative and to promote bowel regularity.

Ingredients: The primary active ingredients in cascara sagrada are anthraquinone glycosides, particularly cascarosides A and B. These compounds stimulate peristalsis in the colon, leading to increased bowel movements.

How to Prepare: Cascara sagrada is typically prepared as an herbal tea, tincture, or capsule. To make tea, dried cascara sagrada bark is steeped in hot water for several minutes before being strained and consumed. Tinctures are prepared by steeping the bark in alcohol to extract its active compounds.

Dosage: The appropriate dosage of cascara sagrada can vary depending on the specific preparation and intended use. It's important to follow the recommended dosage on the product label or consult with a healthcare professional for personalized guidance.

How to Use: Cascara sagrada tea or tincture is typically taken orally. It's important to start with a low dose and gradually increase if needed to avoid potential side effects such as cramping or diarrhea.

Side Effects: Cascara sagrada is considered safe for short-term use when used as directed. However, long-term or excessive use may lead to dependence, electrolyte imbalance, or dehydration. It may also interact with certain medications or have adverse effects in individuals with certain health conditions. It's important to use cascara sagrada under the guidance of a healthcare professional and to discontinue use if any adverse effects occur.

Cell Food:

Definition: Cell Food is a dietary supplement marketed as a highly oxygenating and alkalizing formula. It's claimed to support overall health and vitality by providing essential nutrients and oxygen to the cells.

Ingredients: The exact ingredients of Cell Food can vary depending on the brand, but it typically contains a proprietary blend of minerals, enzymes, electrolytes, and trace elements. Some common ingredients may include purified water, dissolved oxygen, seawater extract, and plant-based enzymes.

How to Prepare: Cell Food is usually available in liquid form and is typically taken orally. It can be consumed directly or diluted in water or juice before consumption.

Dosage: The dosage of Cell Food can vary depending on the specific product and individual needs. It's important to follow the recommended dosage on the product label or consult with a healthcare professional for personalized guidance.

How to Use: Cell Food is typically taken orally, either directly or mixed into water or juice. It's important to shake the bottle well before use and to store it according to the manufacturer's instructions.

Side Effects: Cell Food is generally considered safe for most people when used as directed. However, some individuals may experience mild digestive upset or allergic reactions to certain ingredients. It's essential to consult with a healthcare provider before starting any new supplement regimen, especially if you have underlying health conditions or are taking medications.

Chaparral:

Definition: Chaparral, scientifically known as Larrea tridentata, is a shrub native to the southwestern United States and northern Mexico. It has been used for centuries by Native American tribes for its medicinal properties and is commonly used in herbal medicine today.

Ingredients: Chaparral contains several bioactive compounds, including nordihydroguaiaretic acid (NDGA), flavonoids, lignans, and volatile oils. NDGA is believed to be the primary active compound responsible for many of chaparral's therapeutic effects.

How to Prepare: Chaparral can be prepared and consumed in various forms, including teas, tinctures, capsules, and topical preparations. To make tea, dried chaparral leaves are steeped in hot water for several minutes before being strained and consumed. Tinctures are prepared by steeping the herb in alcohol or vinegar to extract its active compounds.

Dosage: The appropriate dosage of chaparral can vary depending on the specific form and intended use. It's important to follow the recommended dosage on the product label or consult with a healthcare professional for personalized guidance.

How to Use: Chaparral tea or tincture is typically taken orally. It can also be applied topically to the skin for certain conditions. It's important to use chaparral products as directed and to discontinue use if any adverse effects occur.

Side Effects: Chaparral is generally considered safe for most people when used in moderate amounts. However, excessive intake or prolonged use may lead to liver toxicity or other adverse effects. It may also interact with certain medications or have adverse effects in individuals with certain health conditions. It's important to use chaparral under the guidance of a healthcare professional and to discontinue use if any adverse effects occur.

Cocolmeca:

Definition: Cocolmeca, also known as Smilax ornata or sarsaparilla, is a flowering vine native to Mexico and Central America. It has been used traditionally in Mexican and Central American folk medicine for its purported medicinal properties.

Ingredients: Cocolmeca contains various bioactive compounds, including saponins, flavonoids, and plant sterols. These compounds are believed to contribute to the herb's medicinal properties, including its potential as a diuretic, blood purifier, and anti-inflammatory agent.

How to Prepare: Cocolmeca is commonly prepared and consumed as an herbal tea or decoction. To make tea, dried cocolmeca roots or leaves are steeped in hot water for several minutes before being strained and consumed. Decoctions involve boiling the roots or leaves in water to extract their active compounds.

Dosage: The appropriate dosage of cocolmeca can vary depending on factors such as age, health status, and the specific preparation being used. It's important to follow the recommended dosage on the product label or consult with a qualified herbalist or healthcare professional for personalized guidance.

How to Use: Cocolmeca tea or decoction is typically taken orally. It can also be used topically for certain skin conditions. It's important to use cocolmeca products as directed and to discontinue use if any adverse effects occur.

Side Effects: Cocolmeca is generally considered safe for most people when used in moderate amounts. However, excessive intake may lead to digestive upset or other adverse effects. It may also interact with certain medications or have adverse effects in individuals with certain health conditions. It's important to use cocolmeca under the guidance of a healthcare professional and to discontinue use if any adverse effects occur.

Contribo:

Definition: Contribo, also known as Aristolochiatrilobata, is a vine native to the Caribbean and Central America. It has been used traditionally in folk medicine for various purposes, including as a remedy for digestive issues, inflammation, and pain relief.

Ingredients: Contribo contains several bioactive compounds, including aristolochic acids, flavonoids, and alkaloids. These compounds are believed to contribute to the herb's medicinal properties, including its potential as an anti-inflammatory and analgesic agent.

How to Prepare: Contribo is typically prepared and consumed as an herbal tea or decoction. To make tea, dried contribo leaves or stems are steeped in hot water for several minutes before being strained and consumed. Decoctions involve boiling the leaves or stems in water to extract their active compounds.

Dosage: The appropriate dosage of contribo can vary depending on factors such as age, health status, and the specific preparation being used. It's important to follow the recommended dosage on the product label or consult with a qualified herbalist or healthcare professional for personalized guidance.

How to Use: Contribo tea or decoction is typically taken orally. It's important to use contribo products as directed and to discontinue use if any adverse effects occur.

Side Effects: Contribo contains aristolochic acids, which have been associated with serious adverse effects, including kidney damage and cancer. Due to these safety concerns, the use of contribo is highly discouraged, and it's important to avoid products containing aristolochic acids. Individuals should seek alternative remedies for their health needs.

Dandelion Root:

Definition: Dandelion, scientifically known as Taraxacum officinale, is a common flowering plant found worldwide. While often considered a pesky weed, dandelion has a long history of use in traditional medicine for its various health benefits.

Ingredients: Dandelion root contains several bioactive compounds, including sesquiterpene lactones, triterpenes, flavonoids, and polysaccharides. These compounds are believed to contribute to the herb's medicinal properties, including its potential as a diuretic, digestive aid, and liver tonic.

How to Prepare: Dandelion root can be prepared and consumed in various forms, including teas, tinctures, capsules, and extracts. To make tea, dried dandelion root is steeped in hot water for several minutes before being strained and consumed. Tinctures are prepared by steeping the root in alcohol or vinegar to extract its active compounds.

Dosage: The appropriate dosage of dandelion root can vary depending on factors such as age, health status, and the specific preparation being used. It's important to follow the recommended dosage on the product label or consult with a qualified herbalist or healthcare professional for personalized guidance.

How to Use: Dandelion root tea, tincture, or capsules are typically taken orally. It's important to use dandelion root products as directed and to discontinue use if any adverse effects occur.

Side Effects: Dandelion root is generally considered safe for most people when used in moderate amounts. However, some individuals may experience allergic reactions or digestive upset. It may also interact with certain medications or have adverse effects in individuals with certain health conditions. It's important to use dandelion root under the guidance of a healthcare professional and to discontinue use if any adverse effects occur.

Green Food Plus:

Definition: Green Food Plus is a dietary supplement formulated to provide a concentrated source of nutrients derived from various green plants. It's designed to support overall health and well-being by delivering essential vitamins, minerals, antioxidants, and phytonutrients.

Ingredients: Green Food Plus typically contains a blend of powdered green vegetables, grasses, algae, and other plant-based ingredients. Common ingredients may include wheatgrass, barley grass, spirulina, chlorella, alfalfa, kale, spinach, and broccoli, among others.

How to Prepare: Green Food Plus is usually available in powder form and can be mixed with water, juice, or smoothies. It's important to follow the recommended dosage on the product label and to consume it as part of a balanced diet.

Dosage: The appropriate dosage of Green Food Plus can vary depending on the specific product and individual needs. It's important to follow the recommended dosage on the product label or consult with a healthcare professional for personalized guidance.

How to Use: Green Food Plus powder is typically mixed with water, juice, or smoothies and consumed orally. It's often taken once or twice daily, preferably with meals, to maximize nutrient absorption.

Side Effects: Green Food Plus is generally considered safe for most people when used as directed. However, some individuals may experience digestive upset or allergic reactions to certain ingredients. It's important to consult with a healthcare provider before starting any new supplement regimen, especially if you have underlying health conditions or are taking medications.

Guaco:

Definition: Guaco, also known as Mikania cordata or Mikania glomerata, is a medicinal plant native to Central and South America. It has a long history of use in traditional medicine for its potential therapeutic properties.

Ingredients: Guaco contains several bioactive compounds, including coumarins, flavonoids, tannins, and saponins. These compounds are believed to contribute to the herb's medicinal properties, including its potential as an expectorant, anti-inflammatory, and antispasmodic agent.

How to Prepare: Guaco is typically prepared and consumed as an herbal tea or infusion. To make tea, dried guaco leaves are steeped in hot water for several minutes before being strained and consumed.

Dosage: The appropriate dosage of guaco can vary depending on factors such as age, health status, and the specific preparation being used. It's important to follow the recommended dosage on the product label or consult with a qualified herbalist or healthcare professional for personalized guidance.

How to Use: Guaco tea is typically taken orally. It can be consumed on its own or mixed with honey or other herbal teas for added flavor.

Side Effects: Guaco is generally considered safe for most people when used in moderate amounts. However, some individuals may experience allergic reactions or digestive upset. It may also interact with certain medications or have adverse effects in individuals with certain health conditions. It's important to use guaco under the guidance of a healthcare professional and to discontinue use if any adverse effects occur.

Herban Iron:

Definition: Herban Iron is a dietary supplement designed to provide an easily absorbable form of iron to support healthy iron levels in the body. It's particularly beneficial for individuals with iron deficiency or anemia.

Ingredients: Herban Iron typically contains iron in the form of ferrous bisglycinate, which is a highly bioavailable and gentle form of iron that is less likely to cause digestive upset or constipation compared to other forms of iron. It may also contain other ingredients such as vitamin C to enhance iron absorption.

How to Prepare: Herban Iron is usually available in capsule or liquid form. Capsules are taken orally with water, while liquid forms may be mixed with water or juice before consumption. It's important to follow the recommended dosage on the product label.

Dosage: The appropriate dosage of Herban Iron depends on factors such as age, gender, and the severity of iron deficiency. It's important to consult with a healthcare professional to determine the correct dosage for individual needs.

How to Use: Herban Iron capsules are typically taken orally with water, while liquid forms may be mixed with water or juice before consumption. It's important to take Herban Iron as directed and to avoid taking it with dairy products, antacids, or other substances that may interfere with iron absorption.

Side Effects: While Herban Iron is generally considered safe for most people when used as directed, some individuals may experience mild side effects such as gastrointestinal discomfort or constipation. It's important to consult with a healthcare professional before starting any new supplement regimen, especially if you have underlying health conditions or are taking medications.

Blood Purifier:

Definition: Blood purifiers are herbal remedies or dietary supplements believed to cleanse or detoxify the blood, often promoting overall health and well-being. They are thought to support the body's natural detoxification processes and improve blood circulation.

Ingredients: Blood purifiers may contain a variety of herbs and botanical extracts known for their purported cleansing and detoxifying properties. Common ingredients include burdock root, red clover, dandelion root, and yellow dock root, among others.

How to Prepare: Blood purifiers are typically available in various forms, including capsules, tablets, powders, and liquid extracts. They are usually taken orally with water or juice, following the recommended dosage on the product label.

Dosage: The dosage of blood purifiers can vary depending on the specific product and individual needs. It's important to adhere to the recommended dosage on the product label or consult with a healthcare professional for personalized guidance.

How to Use: Blood purifiers are typically taken orally, either with water or mixed into beverages. They are often used as part of a detoxification regimen or to support overall health and vitality.

Side Effects: While blood purifiers are generally considered safe for most people when used as directed, some individuals may experience side effects such as digestive discomfort, allergic reactions, or interactions with medications. It's important to consult with a healthcare provider before starting any new supplement regimen, especially if you have underlying health conditions or are taking medications.

Blue Vervain:

Definition: Blue vervain, also known as Verbena hastata, is a perennial herb native to North America. It has been used in traditional medicine for centuries to treat various ailments, including anxiety, insomnia, and digestive issues.

Ingredients: Blue vervain contains several active compounds, including aucubin, verbenalin, and volatile oils. These compounds are believed to contribute to the herb's medicinal properties.

How to Prepare: Blue vervain is typically consumed as a tea or tincture. To make tea, dried blue vervain leaves and flowers are steeped in hot water for several minutes before being strained and consumed. Tinctures are prepared by steeping the herb in alcohol or vinegar to extract its active compounds.

Dosage: The appropriate dosage of blue vervain can vary depending on factors such as age, health status, and the specific preparation being used. It's important to follow the recommended dosage on the product label or consult with a qualified herbalist or healthcare professional for personalized guidance.

How to Use: Blue vervain tea or tincture is typically taken orally. It can be consumed on its own or mixed with honey or other herbal teas for added flavor.

Side Effects: While blue vervain is generally considered safe for most people when used in moderation, excessive intake may cause digestive upset or allergic reactions in some individuals. Pregnant or breastfeeding women should avoid blue vervain due to its potential to stimulate uterine contractions. As with any herbal remedy, it's important to consult with a healthcare provider before using blue vervain, especially if you have underlying health conditions or are taking medications.

Bromide Plus Powder:

Definition: Bromide Plus Powder is a dietary supplement formulated to support thyroid health and promote overall well-being. It typically contains a blend of herbs and minerals that are believed to have beneficial effects on thyroid function.

Ingredients: Bromide Plus Powder often contains a combination of herbs such as bladderwrack, sea moss, and burdock root, along with minerals like iodine and potassium phosphate. These ingredients are thought to support thyroid function and maintain optimal iodine levels in the body.

How to Prepare: Bromide Plus Powder is usually mixed with water or juice to create a drinkable solution. It's important to follow the instructions on the product label for dosage and preparation.

Dosage: The dosage of Bromide Plus Powder can vary depending on the specific product and individual needs. It's crucial to consult with a healthcare professional or follow the recommended dosage on the product label to avoid potential side effects.

How to Use: Bromide Plus Powder is typically taken orally by mixing the recommended dosage with water or juice. It's important to shake or stir the mixture well before consuming it to ensure even distribution of the ingredients.

Side Effects: While Bromide Plus Powder is generally considered safe when used as directed, some individuals may experience side effects such as digestive discomfort or allergic reactions to certain ingredients. It's essential to consult with a healthcare provider before starting any new supplement regimen, especially if you have underlying health conditions or are taking medications.

Bugleweed:

Definition: Bugleweed, also known as Lycopusvirginicus, is a perennial herb native to North America and Europe. It has been used in traditional medicine to treat various conditions, including hyperthyroidism, anxiety, and insomnia.

Ingredients: Bugleweed contains several active compounds, including lithospermic acid, phenolic acids, and flavonoids. These compounds are believed to contribute to the herb's medicinal properties, particularly its ability to regulate thyroid function.

How to Prepare: Bugleweed is commonly consumed as a tea or tincture. To make tea, dried bugleweed leaves and flowers are steeped in hot water for several minutes before being strained and consumed. Tinctures are prepared by steeping the herb in alcohol or vinegar to extract its active compounds.

Dosage: The appropriate dosage of bugleweed can vary depending on factors such as age, health status, and the specific preparation being used. It's important to follow the recommended dosage on the product label or consult with a qualified herbalist or healthcare professional for personalized guidance.

How to Use: Bugleweed tea or tincture is typically taken orally. It can be consumed on its own or mixed with honey or other herbal teas for added flavor.

Side Effects: While bugleweed is generally considered safe for most people when used in moderation, excessive intake may cause digestive upset or allergic reactions in some individuals.

Pregnant or breastfeeding women should avoid bugleweed due to its potential to stimulate uterine contractions. As with any herbal remedy, it's important to consult with a healthcare provider before using bugleweed, especially if you have underlying health conditions or are taking medications.

Hops:

Definition: Hops, scientifically known as Humulus lupulus, is a perennial climbing vine native to Europe, Asia, and North America. It is primarily known for its use in brewing beer but has also been used historically in traditional medicine for its potential health benefits.

Ingredients: Hops flowers contain various bioactive compounds, including bitter acids (such as humulone and lupulone), essential oils, flavonoids, and polyphenols. These compounds are believed to contribute to the herb's medicinal properties, including its potential as a sedative, relaxant, and digestive aid.

How to Prepare: Hops is typically consumed as an herbal tea, tincture, or in supplement form (such as capsules or tablets). To make tea, dried hops flowers are steeped in hot water for several minutes before being strained and consumed.

Dosage: The appropriate dosage of hops can vary depending on factors such as age, health status, and the specific preparation being used. It's important to follow the recommended dosage on the product label or consult with a qualified herbalist or healthcare professional for personalized guidance.

How to Use: Hops tea, tincture, or supplements are typically taken orally. It's often used to promote relaxation, relieve anxiety, and support sleep.

Side Effects: Hops is generally considered safe for most people when used in moderate amounts. However, some individuals may experience mild side effects such as drowsiness, gastrointestinal upset, or allergic reactions. It may also interact with certain medications or have adverse effects in individuals with certain health conditions, such as depression or hormone-sensitive conditions. It's important to use hops under the guidance of a healthcare professional and to discontinue use if any adverse effects occur.

Kelp:

Definition: Kelp refers to several species of large brown algae belonging to the Laminariales order. It is commonly found in underwater forests along rocky coastlines around the world. Kelp has been used for centuries in various cultures, particularly in East Asia, for its nutritional and medicinal properties.

Ingredients: Kelp is rich in various nutrients, including iodine, vitamins (such as vitamin K, vitamin C, and B vitamins), minerals (including calcium, magnesium, and potassium), antioxidants, and fiber. These nutrients are believed to contribute to the seaweed's potential health benefits, including its role in thyroid function, bone health, and immune support.

How to Prepare: Kelp is typically consumed dried, powdered, or in supplement form (such as capsules or tablets). It can also be used in cooking, particularly in soups, salads, and stir-fries. Kelp supplements are available in various forms, including powdered extracts, tablets, and liquid extracts.

Dosage: The appropriate dosage of kelp can vary depending on factors such as age, health status, and the specific preparation being used. It's important to follow the recommended dosage on the product label or consult with a qualified healthcare professional for personalized guidance.

How to Use: Kelp supplements are typically taken orally with water. They can be consumed as part of a daily nutritional regimen to support overall health and well-being. Kelp can also be incorporated into recipes as a flavorful and nutritious ingredient.

Side Effects: While kelp is generally considered safe for most people when consumed in moderate amounts, excessive intake of iodine-rich foods or supplements, including kelp, can lead to thyroid dysfunction or iodine toxicity. Some individuals may also be allergic to seaweed and experience allergic reactions. Pregnant or breastfeeding individuals should consult with a healthcare professional before using kelp supplements. It's important to use kelp under the guidance of a healthcare professional and to discontinue use if any adverse effects occur.

Ginseng:

Definition: Ginseng refers to several species of perennial plants belonging to the Panax genus, including Panax ginseng (Asian ginseng) and Panax quinquefolius (American ginseng). Ginseng has been used for centuries in traditional medicine, particularly in East Asia, for its potential health benefits.

Ingredients: Ginseng root contains various bioactive compounds, including ginsenosides, polysaccharides, and peptides. These compounds are believed to contribute to the herb's medicinal properties, including its potential as an adaptogen, immune enhancer, and cognitive booster.

How to Prepare: Ginseng is typically consumed as a powdered root, herbal tea, tincture, or in supplement form (such as capsules or tablets). To make tea, dried ginseng root slices are simmered in water for several minutes before being strained and consumed.

Dosage: The appropriate dosage of ginseng can vary depending on factors such as age, health status, and the specific preparation being used. It's important to follow the recommended dosage on the product label or consult with a qualified herbalist or healthcare professional for personalized guidance.

How to Use: Ginseng powder, tea, tincture, or supplements are typically taken orally. It's often used to support energy levels, enhance cognitive function, and promote overall well-being.

Side Effects: Ginseng is generally considered safe for most people when used in moderate amounts. However, some individuals may experience mild side effects such as insomnia, gastrointestinal upset, or headaches. It may also interact with certain medications or have adverse effects in individuals with certain health conditions, such as high blood pressure or diabetes. Pregnant or breastfeeding individuals should consult with a healthcare professional before using ginseng supplements. It's important to use ginseng under the guidance of a healthcare professional and to discontinue use if any adverse effects occur.

Goldenseal:

Definition: Goldenseal, scientifically known as Hydrastis canadensis, is a perennial herb native to North America. It has a long history of use in traditional Native American medicine and later in folk medicine for its potential health benefits.

Ingredients: Goldenseal root contains various bioactive compounds, including alkaloids (such as berberine and hydrastine), flavonoids, and volatile oils. These compounds are believed to contribute to the herb's medicinal properties, including its potential as an antimicrobial, anti-inflammatory, and immune enhancer.

How to Prepare: Goldenseal is typically consumed as an herbal tea, tincture, or in supplement form (such as capsules or tablets). To make tea, dried goldenseal root or leaves are steeped in hot water for several minutes before being strained and consumed.

Dosage: The appropriate dosage of goldenseal can vary depending on factors such as age, health status, and the specific preparation being used. It's important to follow the recommended dosage on the product label or consult with a qualified herbalist or healthcare professional for personalized guidance.

How to Use: Goldenseal tea, tincture, or supplements are typically taken orally. It's often used to support immune function, promote digestive health, and soothe inflammation.

Side Effects: Goldenseal is generally considered safe for most people when used in moderate amounts. However, some individuals may experience mild side effects such as gastrointestinal upset or allergic reactions. It may also interact with certain medications or have adverse effects in individuals with certain health conditions, such as high blood pressure or pregnancy. It's important to use goldenseal under the guidance of a healthcare professional and to discontinue use if any adverse effects occur.

THE END

www.ingramcontent.com/pod-product-compliance
Lightning Source LLC
Chambersburg PA
CBHW080638280726
48659CB00025BA/2523